Fibre

by Jane Inglis

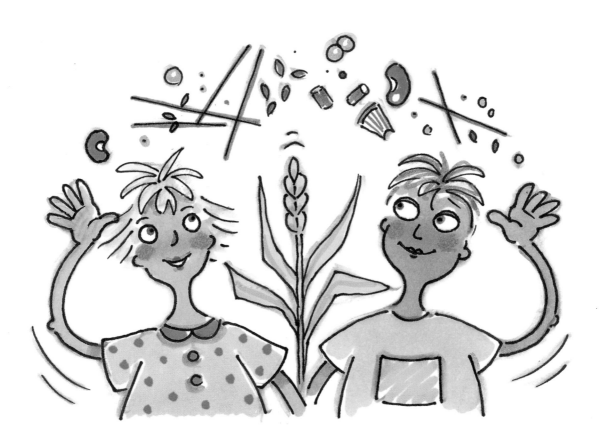

Wayland

Additives
Vitamins
Fibre
Sugar
Fats
Proteins

Words printed in **bold** can be found in the glossary on page 30.

First published in 1992 by Wayland (Publishers) Ltd.
61 Western Road, Hove, East Sussex, BN3 1JD

British Library Cataloguing in Publication Data

Inglis, Jane
  Fibre. – (Food Facts Series)
  I. Title II. Jackson, Maureen
  III. Yates, John IV. Series
  641.1
  ISBN 0 7502 0393 5

Series Editor: Kathryn Smith
Designer: Helen White
Artwork: John Yates
Cartoons: Maureen Jackson

Typesetting by White Design
Printed and bound in Belgium by Casterman S.A.

Contents

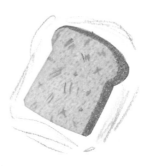

What is fibre ?

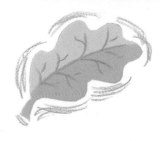

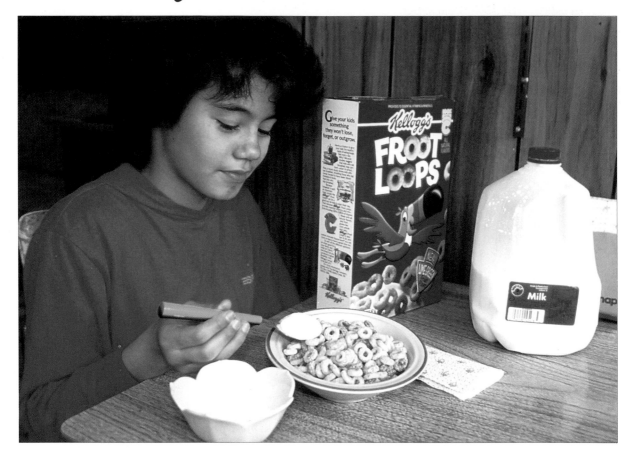

What is fibre? A fibre is a fine thread. The word fibre is also used for things made of fine threads, like cloth. This book is about dietary fibre, or the fibre that we eat. Most of our food is **digested** and used to keep our bodies fit and healthy, and to give us energy. But the rest of our food is not digested. It passes right through the body and leaves it as waste.

ABOVE How healthy is the food you eat?

RIGHT These high-fibre foods are made using unrefined ingredients; nothing has been added or taken away.

Fibre is the name of something found only in plants, which is not digested but passes right through the body and helps the **digestive system** to work well. If you look at high-fibre foods (foods containing a lot of fibre) under a strong magnifying glass or a **microscope** you can see the threads that give dietary fibre its name.

All living things are made up of millions of tiny **cells**. The cells of the plants we use for food are like parcels wrapped in fibre. Inside the cells are **nutrients** that nourish us; outside are the cell walls made up of fibre. They help to make plants stand up, rather like the bony skeletons of animals.

Meat contains no fibre. Nor do dairy products or any other foods that come from animals. Some fruit and vegetables contain a lot; others, such as strawberries, contain less.

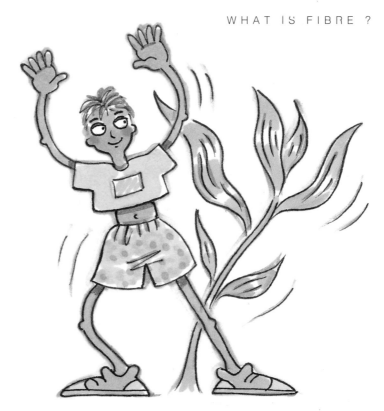

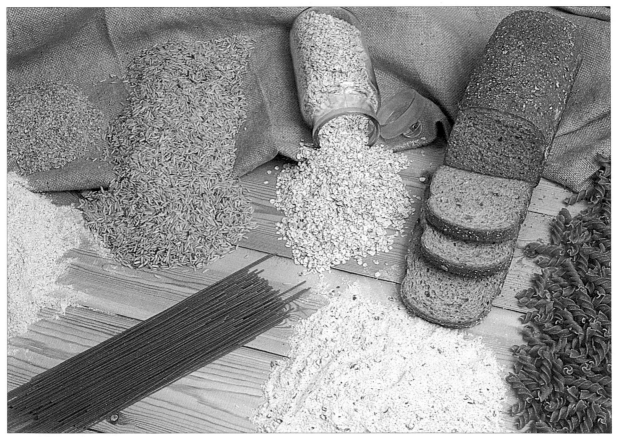

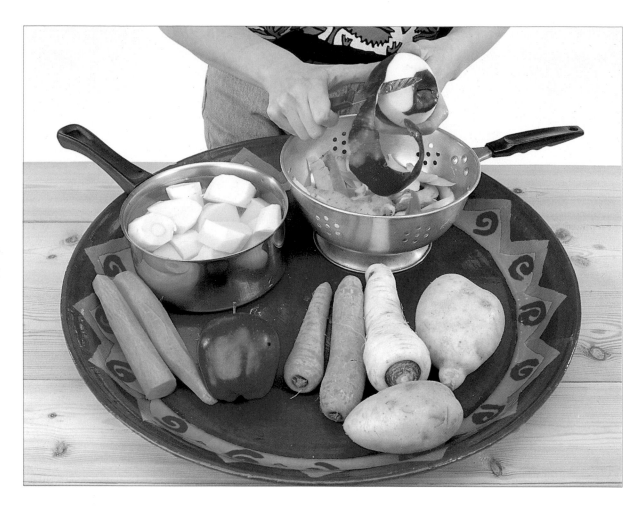

ABOVE Peeling vegetables not only removes a lot of their fibre; it also removes many of the valuable vitamins and minerals which are stored just beneath the skin.

Cereals in their natural form, (that is whole grains such as brown rice, whole-wheat flakes and oats) are a particularly good source of fibre.

There is more fibre on the outside of nuts, fruit, peas and beans, than on the inside. Much of it is lost when the outside layer is taken away. This is what happens when fruit and vegetables are peeled, white flour is milled, sugar is **extracted** from sugar beet or cane, and oil is pressed from nuts and seeds. We keep and use the part of the plant that contains most of the nutrients. Often the rest – the peel, skins, and husks – is thrown away or used to feed farm animals.

Foods which have been treated like this are called refined, or processed foods. We now know that the fibre in the tough outer parts of the plants we use for food is a very important part of our **diet**.

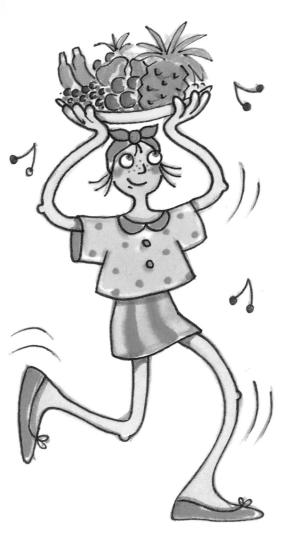

own skin all around it, so these fruits have more fibre than single berries. They take longer to chew, too, than low-fibre fruit (fruit containing little fibre) like strawberries.

Different kinds of fibre are found in different plants, but they are all good for our health. This book explains why this is so, why so many of us do not eat enough fibre, and how you can increase the amount in your diet.

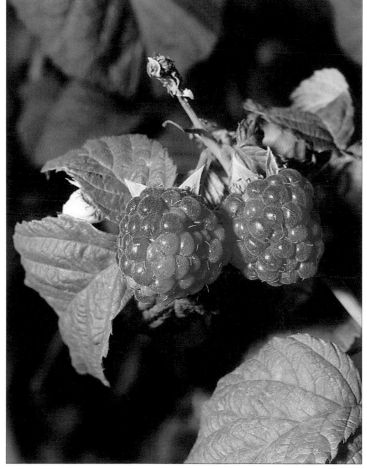

If we throw it away or feed it to farm animals we are wasting it. The refined diet we are left with is bad for our health.

Raspberries and black-berries are also very high in fibre. This will not surprise you if you remember that the outsides of fruits contain more fibre than the insides. Look closely at a raspberry or blackberry. Each fruit is made up of lots of tiny pieces, joined together. Each piece has its

Science Corner

We cannot always tell by looking at food, or even by eating it, whether it contains a lot of fibre. But chewy foods that take quite a while to eat are usually high in fibre. Have a close look at some dried figs, prunes and apricots. All of these contain a lot of fibre. Cut them open and look at them through a magnifying glass, or better still a microscope. Feel the **texture** with your fingers. You should be able to see and feel lots of tiny threads, and seeds in the figs as well.

After cutting up the dried fruit, wash and eat it. Figs, prunes and apricots are all sweet and tasty. It takes quite a long time to chew your way through them. Their texture, and the time it takes to eat them, are clues to the large amount of fibre they contain.

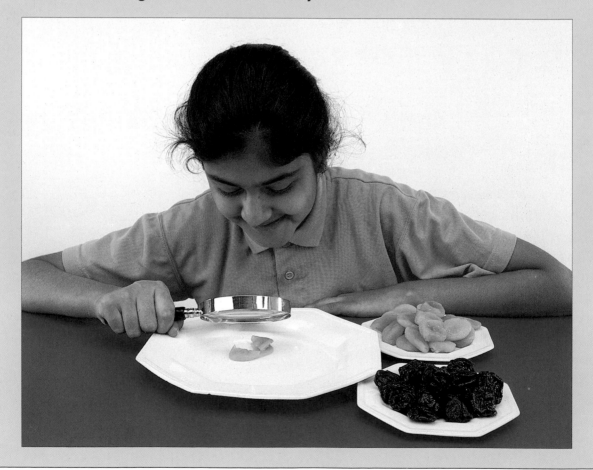

The history of fibre

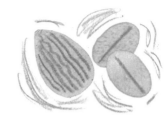

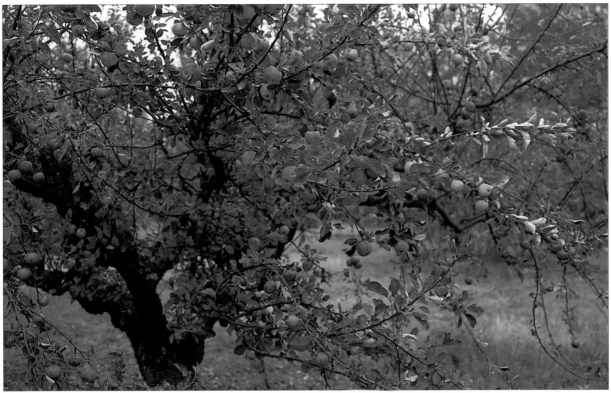

The food our early **ancestors** ate must have contained a lot of fibre, but finding and eating it would have been very hard work. Before the days of farming groups of people lived by roaming around the land, gathering wild plants to eat and hunting animals. Most of their food came from plants, so people must have spent much of their time searching for the right plants, preparing and eating them.

ABOVE This tree is heavily laden with apples. These days many people buy their groceries from a supermarket. It is easy to forget where the food actually comes from, and that nature provides everything we need for a healthy diet.

The wild grass seeds, nuts, berries and other fruits they ate were all smaller than those we eat today, and contained more fibre. It must have taken a very long time to remove all the parts they couldn't eat and to chew the rest enough to make it edible.

Once people started to grow crops, in the Stone Age, they lived very different lives and the way they ate began to change a lot too.

Investigation

You can find out what this early way of life was like if you spend a day in the countryside in autumn. Would you survive if you had to live without modern food? Make a list of the fruits and nuts you know are safe to eat. Do not take risks with unknown berries: some of them are **poisonous.** So are some mushrooms. You probably didn't put grass seeds on your list, because seeds of our wild grasses are very small. But they are also very nourishing. Do you think you would have enough to eat in order to survive?

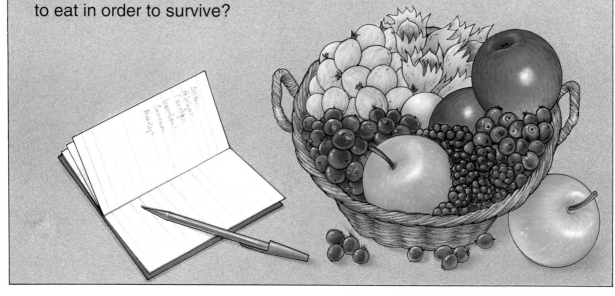

People started to grow cereal grains for food. These specially grown grains were bigger and provided more food, but they probably contained less fibre. People stayed in one place, and began to grind the grains with stones instead of with their teeth. Early millstones have been found at many places where Stone Age people lived.

Stone Age mills, or querns, were big round stones worked by hand. A hole through the middle of the top stone allowed the grain to fall through on to a flat stone underneath. The top stone was turned by hand and the grain was crushed between the two. Flour made in this way contained just as much fibre as the whole grain. Nothing was removed.

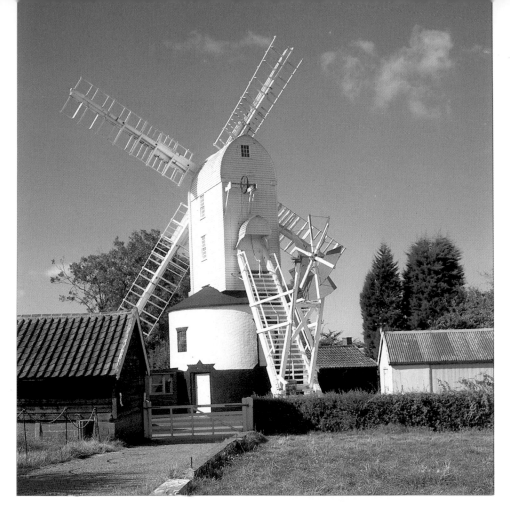

LEFT Windmills use the wind to move their sails. This creates the power to turn the millstones inside the mill and grind the grain into flour.

BELOW The inside of a working water mill. Outside, a huge wheel is turned by falling water in order to create the power to work the mill.

Through the ages many different ways were found to make milling easier. Animals and the power of wind and water were all used in different ways to turn the millstones.

The colour of bread made with these whole flours was always brownish, and the bread was heavy in texture. In the past **yeasts** (used to make bread rise) were not as good as the ones we use today, so bread was often tough and doughy. It was full of fibre and very nourishing, but sometimes quite hard to eat.

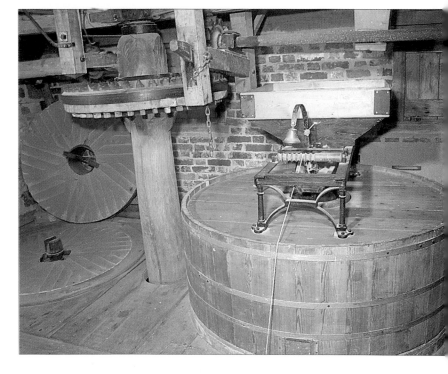

BELOW *This tasty sandwich made with wholemeal bread contains at least twice as much fibre as the same sandwich made with white bread.*

White bread

We know that as long ago as ancient Egyptian and Roman times, bread was made to look whiter for rich people to eat. This was done in all sorts of ways. Sometimes white powders, such as chalk, were added. Sometimes flour was sifted through **papyrus sieves** (in ancient Egypt) or layers of cloth (in ancient Rome) to take out the cases of the grain.

This must have taken a very long time, and most people could not afford to buy this kind of bread. It was not as pale as the white bread we eat today because not all of the fibre could be removed by sieving. It was a **luxury** food for the wealthy. Most people continued to eat dark whole-meal bread which was actually more healthy because it contained a lot of fibre.

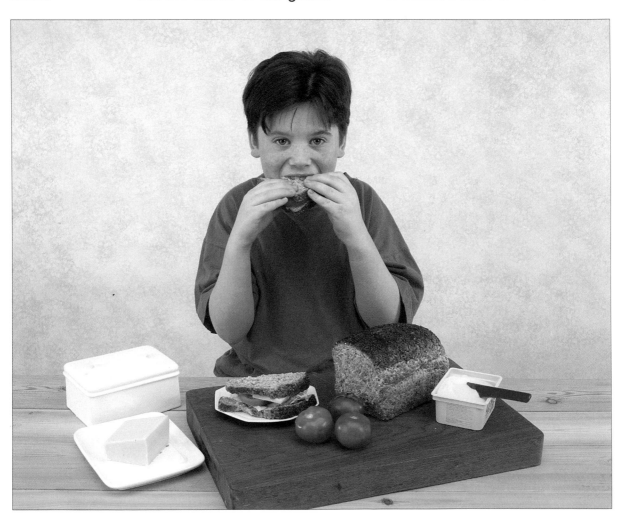

Refined flour

It was not until the **Industrial Revolution** in the nineteenth century that a large-scale method was invented to make white flour. Before then flour had been milled using stones, and had taken a long time. Now new roller mills were built. These were cheap, fast and efficient. It was possible to separate all the wheat germ and husk from the flour, which was therefore very white and kept well. Instead of being a luxury for the rich, white bread was now cheap enough for everyone.

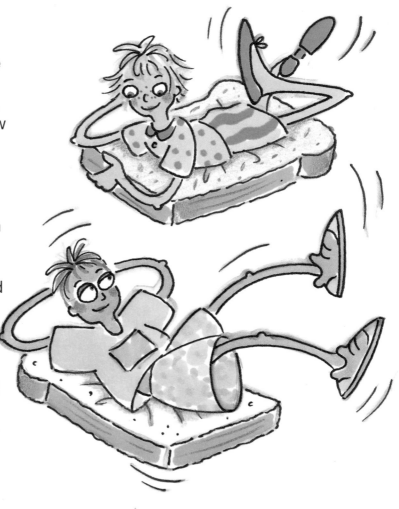

Unfortunately this meant that the diet of poor people, who had always eaten a lot of bread because it was cheap, suddenly lost a lot of its good-ness. Vitamins and minerals were all lost from the grain in this method of removing the husk and germ.

White flour is only one example of a refined food. Many other crops now go straight from the field where they were grown to a factory. Here they are separated by machines into the parts used for human food and the left-overs.

White sugar is made from sugar beet or cane. Much of the bulky waste material left over from making the sugar is fed to animals. Rice, the main food of millions of people in the Far East, is usually polish-ed to remove the outer layer. Whenever food is treated like this, fibre is one of the most important things to be lost.

Science Corner

You can see for yourself all the different things contained in a grain of wheat. Ask an adult to cut one in half. Look closely at the insides of the grain using a magnifying glass. Make a diagram of what you can see. It should look rather like the one below. Can you label the different parts of your drawing, using this diagram to help you?

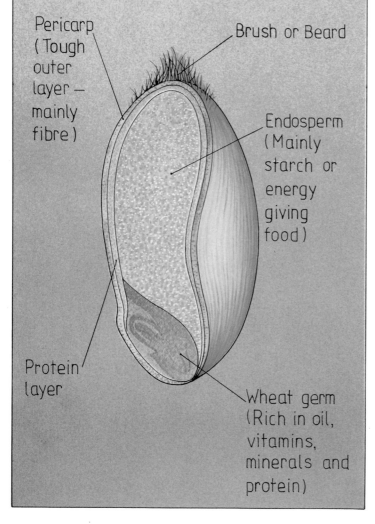

Pericarp (Tough outer layer — mainly fibre)

Brush or Beard

Endosperm (Mainly starch or energy giving food)

Protein layer

Wheat germ (Rich in oil, vitamins, minerals and protein)

When you see how much goodness is wasted when food is refined or processed, you start to wonder why anyone would choose to eat this kind of food. There are several reasons. Freshly-grown food, straight from the garden or field, is much better for us. But most people now live in towns, far from the fields where food is grown. Rich countries can afford to import food grown all over the world. It has to last a long time between harvest and table, and fresh food rots quickly. Once it is processed or refined, food lasts longer. For example, wholemeal flour contains oil from the germ of the wheat, but oil goes bad quickly. White flour, which has had this oil removed during refining, lasts much longer.

People in our modern world have got used to eating food that does not take long to prepare. Refined food is quicker to cook than whole grains, fresh fruit, and vegetables. Also, food manufacturers make much more money out of ready-made meals that have been processed, than from selling whole foods. To prove this, look at a packet of potato crisps. The weight of the bag

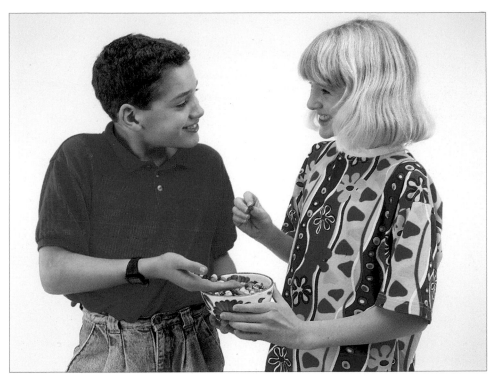

LEFT Nuts and raisins make a delicious snack and are a healthy alternative to sweets and crisps.

will be printed on the outside of the packet. How much would the same weight of potatoes cost if you bought them from a greengrocer? Your answer will be a tiny sum of money, compared to what you paid for the crisps, which have had their skins (containing lots of fibre) removed, and salt, fat and chemical flavouring added.

Advertising helps to persuade people that this is the kind of food they want. Once you are used to a particular kind of food, it takes time and effort to change your eating habits.

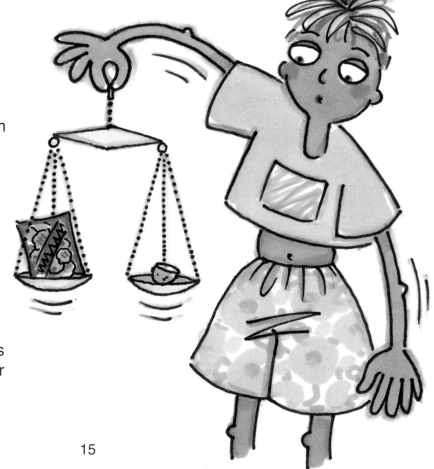

Recipe
Use this recipe to make your own wholemeal bread. It is easy to make, delicious to eat and, of course, full of fibre. Make sure there is an adult present when you are cooking.

Ingredients
1.5 kg wholemeal flour
(if possible **organically** grown)
1 tablespoon of salt

60 g fresh yeast or 30 g dried yeast
1 tablespoon of honey
1 litre lukewarm water

Equipment
large mixing bowl
measuring jug
tablespoon

wooden spoon
3 x 1 kg loaf tins

Method
1. Place the wholemeal flour in a bowl and add the tablespoon of salt.
2. Mix the yeast into half of the lukewarm water, along with the honey (the water should be the same temperature as your finger – dip to test).
3. When the liquid begins to bubble, make a well in the middle of the flour and begin to mix the yeast and water in.
4. Add the rest of the water (at the same temperature), a little at a time as you **knead** the dough. It should be spongy, but not wet.
5. Leave the dough in a warm place, in a bowl, until it doubles in size. Then knead it again for a few minutes.
6. Divide the dough between three greased loaf tins and bake in the top of the oven at 350°C / gas mark 7 for 35-40 minutes. When they are cooked the loaves should sound hollow if you tap them.

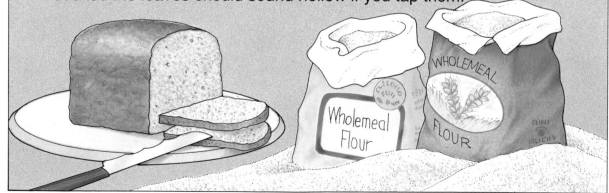

Why is fibre good for you?

This diagram shows the human digestive system. All the food we eat passes through this long, complicated tube. Most of what we eat is **absorbed** and used to repair the body, keep it healthy, and to give us energy. But we cannot use up every bit of our food, so part of the job of the digestive system is to get rid of the waste.

Digestion starts in the mouth, where food makes saliva flow and where chewing breaks it into smaller pieces which can be swallowed. It goes down the throat into the stomach. This is the storage area where strong juices set to work. They break down the food and churn it into a smooth paste.

In the wall of the stomach are muscles that squeeze the paste into the small intestine. Here the food is broken down by more juices into tiny **particles** small enough to pass through the walls of the intestine. They are then carried by the blood to every part of the body to be used for repair work and growth.

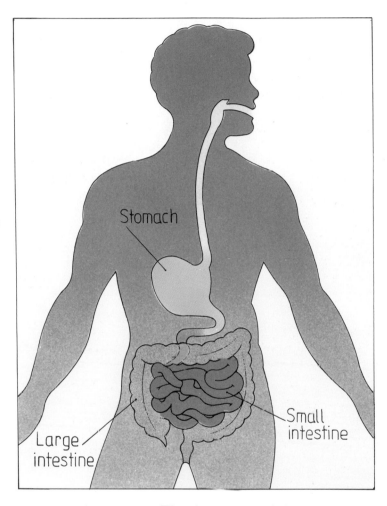

The last part of the tube is called the large intestine. By the time food arrives here, most of what the body can use has been digested. The rest is waste, and the sooner the body gets rid of it, the better. It is no longer any use and, like everything that was once alive,

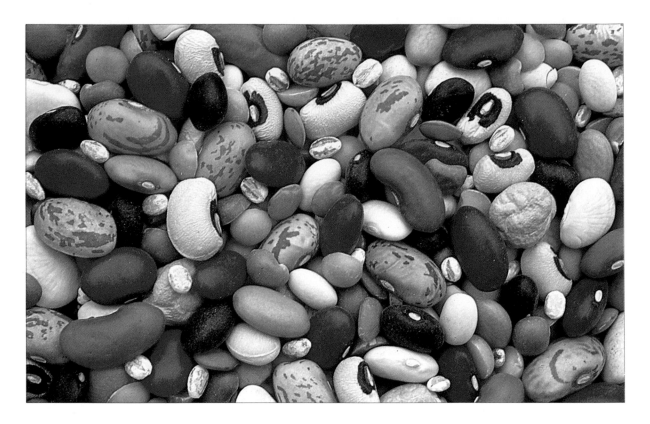

ABOVE Eating beans and pulses is a wonderful way to increase the fibre content of your diet. Beans don't have to be boring; the variety of shapes, colours and tastes is amazing!

it will rot. This would produce **poisons** which would harm the body.

The end of the tube is the storage area for waste called the rectum. The hole through which the waste material leaves the body is called the anus. Our system for getting rid of waste is very good. When enough bulk has piled up in the rectum we feel a need to go to the toilet, where a healthy person will pass a soft, bulky lump of solid waste (doctors call it a stool) at least once a day. This is called excretion.

People who have a high-fibre diet are much less likely to become **constipated** than those who eat lots of refined foods. People who eat lots of fibre will be able to digest their food and get rid of their waste quickly and easily.

Scientists measure the transit time for different types of diet. This means the time it takes from eating a meal to getting rid of the waste material from it. The transit time is longer for refined foods than for foods which contain a lot of fibre. A short transit time is best because there is less chance of poisons from the waste harming the body.

There are huge differences in transit time for groups of people in different parts of the world. People living in villages in **developing countries** have a transit time of about one and a half days. For healthy young people in **developed countries** it is about three days. In some elderly people the transit time may be over two weeks.

Why do people from villages in, for example, Africa take a day and a half to digest their food, while some old people in Britain take two weeks?

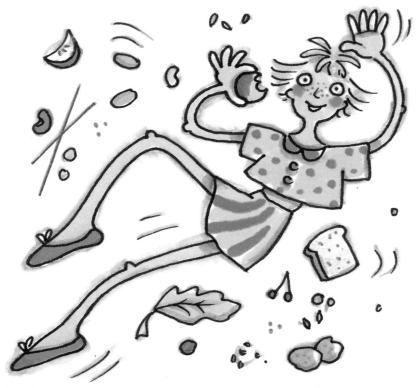

LEFT Try to make sure you do at least half an hour of exercise each day. This will help your digestive system to work more efficiently.

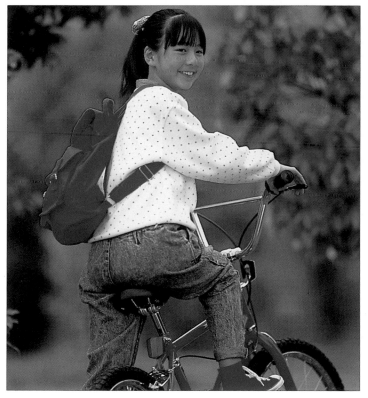

The answer lies in the different ways of life, and most of all in the different diets. Country people from the developing world eat very high-fibre diets; they grow their own food or buy it from the grower; they process it very little and eat mainly unrefined vegetables and cereals. As long as there is enough food, this is much healthier than the normal diet in a developed country.

In rich countries many people eat lots of meat and other animal products containing no fibre at all. The cereals they eat are mainly refined and have lost a great deal of their fibre. Much of their food is grown a long way from where they live. It has been through many **factory processes** that remove fibre as well as other nutrients.

BELOW This meal of curry, rice and chopped vegetables contains most of the ingredients necessary for a healthy diet.

There are other reasons for the longer transit time in rich countries. Elderly people often take less exercise than young adults. This is bad for their digestion as well as for their general health. Anyone with a transit time of two weeks probably sits in a chair all day long and eats nothing but refined foods, with almost no fibre.

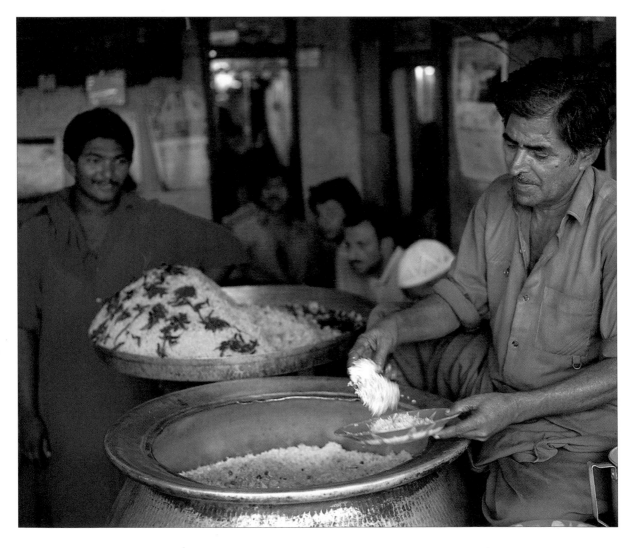

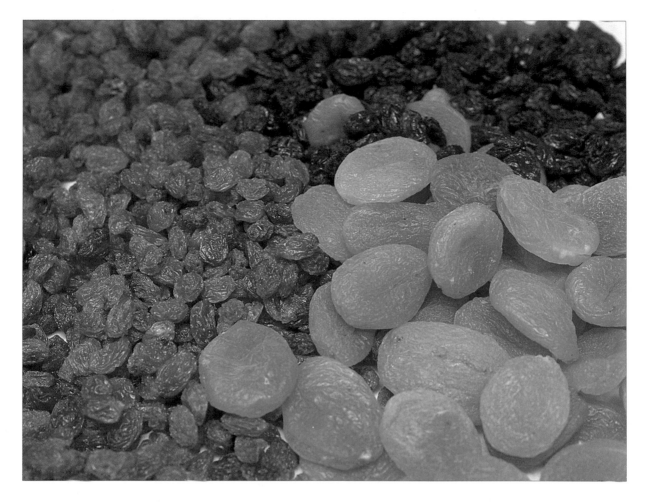

Digestion problems

A person who has only eaten low-fibre food for many years will probably be constipated. But digestive problems over many years can help to cause serious illnesses, as well as constipation. Cancer of the bowel, a killer disease, is almost unknown among people from villages in the developing world, who live on high-fibre diets. It is much more common in the Western world.

ABOVE Dried fruits such as these sweet-tasting currants, sultanas and apricots are particularly high in fibre, and a good way of filling an empty corner between meals.

A high-fibre diet is also less likely to cause our teeth to decay. It is more difficult to over-eat this kind of food. Because it is bulky, it fills the stomach and makes us feel satisfied for longer than refined food. People who want to lose weight find high-fibre foods very useful, but all of us would be healthier eating this way. Changing our diet to include more fibre is easier than you might think.

How to increase the fibre in your diet

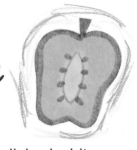

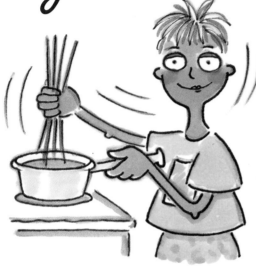

Instead of polished white rice, choose brown. It takes longer to cook but tastes much better. Most supermarkets now sell wholemeal pasta as well as the usual white kinds. Ask whoever does the shopping in your home if you can switch to wholemeal flour in baking. Pastry, biscuits and cakes are all delicious made with whole-meal flour, and of course the fibre level goes zooming up!

BELOW These mouth-watering vegetable burgers have been made using high-fibre ingredients.

When scientists first realized how important fibre was, people began to add **bran** to their food as a quick way of eating more fibre. Bran has more fibre than any other food. But it is quite hard to eat a lot of bran, and not much fun! It is much better to eat your fibre in its natural form than to add bran.

This means swapping refined foods, which have had most of their fibre removed, for unrefined foods. Instead of white bread, try eating wholemeal (always check the food label on bread, as some brown breads may have had some of the fibre removed).

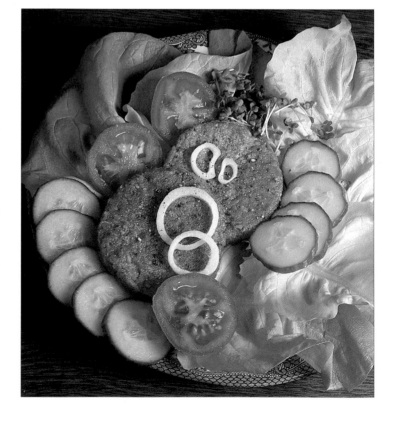

Recipe

Why not try this tasty recipe for brown rice pilaff. It is quick to make, tasty and full of fibre. Make sure there is an adult present when you are cooking.

Ingredients

bunch of spring onions
1 small onion
1 red pepper
1 green pepper
100 g mushrooms
1 carrot

150 g brown rice
2 teaspoons oil
2 teaspoons butter
salt and pepper
½ litre of water

Equipment

non-stick frying pan
wooden spoon
knife

Method

1. Chop the vegetables into very small pieces.
2. Fry the chopped vegetables in the oil and butter for about five minutes. Add the salt and pepper.
3. Add the rice and fry for one minute. Pour on ½ litre of water and leave to simmer slowly for forty minutes, until all the water is absorbed.
4. You can add bits of cooked meat or chicken, if you wish. It is now ready to serve.

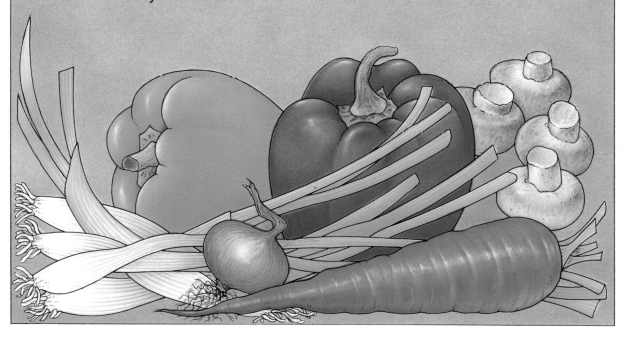

A high-fibre diet also means eating lots of fruit and vegetables and fewer animal products, such as meat and cheese (if you fill up on foods with no fibre, you won't want to eat the high-fibre ones). If you are worried about eating fewer animal products, which contain a lot of **protein** (the body-building food you need to grow) try dried peas and beans. They contain a lot of protein and plenty of fibre too.

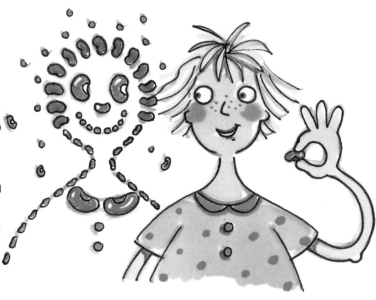

LEFT Soya beans are often used as an alternative to meat because, weight for weight, they contain as much protein as steak and are also high in fibre.

Increasing the amount of fibre you eat means swapping canned drinks and fruit juices, which contain no fibre at all, for raw fresh fruit and drinking water instead. It means eating fruit and nuts for a snack, which contain a lot of fibre, instead of chocolate and sweets .

Where to find your fibre

Cereals which have not been refined or processed are very high in fibre. So are peas, beans and lentils (the family of foods called pulses). Dried fruit contains a lot of fibre and so do vegetables like spinach, although lettuce does not.

BELOW Be creative when you are deciding what to eat. This huge sandwich not only contains a good amount of fibre and other important nutrients; it also looks and tastes appetizing.

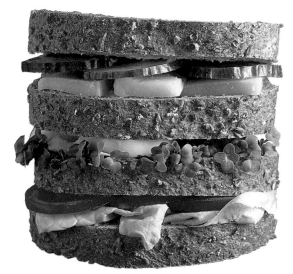

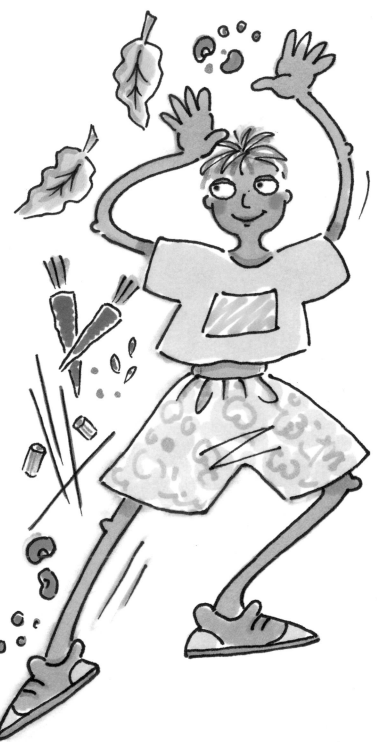

Fresh fruits vary too: blackcurrants and raspberries are high in fibre; strawberries and oranges quite low. As long as you wash fruit and vegetables well, or buy organically-grown ones which have not been sprayed, it is better to eat the skins too, as these contain a lot of fibre.

The table on the next page lists some common foods. It tells you how much fibre there is in 100 g of each one. This is important to know if you are trying to increase the amount of fibre you eat. You also need to think about how much of each food you want to eat. Potatoes do not contain very large amounts of fibre in each 100 g but we eat them so often and in such large quantities, that they are a good way to get fibre.

Almonds contain seven times as much fibre in each 100 g as potatoes, but we don't often eat more than a few almonds at once.

Amount of fibre in 100g of some foods

Food	Fibre	Food	Fibre
Almonds	14·3g	Fried egg	0· g
Apples	1·5g	Grapefruit	0·6g
Apricots (dried)	24·0g	Muesli (average mixture)	7·4g
Bacon	0· g	Oranges	1·5g
Baked beans	7·3g	Pasta (white)	0· g
Bran	44·0g	Pasta (wholemeal)	10· g
Bread (white)	2·7g	Potatoes (cooked in skin)	2·5g
Bread (wholemeal)	8·5g	Raspberries	7·4g
Cornflakes	1· g	Sausages	0· g
		Weetabix	12·7g

Investigation

Look at these two breakfasts.
Which one do you think is more healthy and why?
Use the list on page 26 to help you decide.

Breakfast One
Orange juice
Fried egg, bacon and sausage
Two slices white toast with butter
and marmalade
(Average portions of this breakfast
would contain about 2 g of fibre)

Breakfast Two
Half grapefruit
Weetabix or muesli with yoghurt
Two slices wholemeal toast with
raspberry jam
(Average portions of this breakfast
would contain about 12 g of fibre)

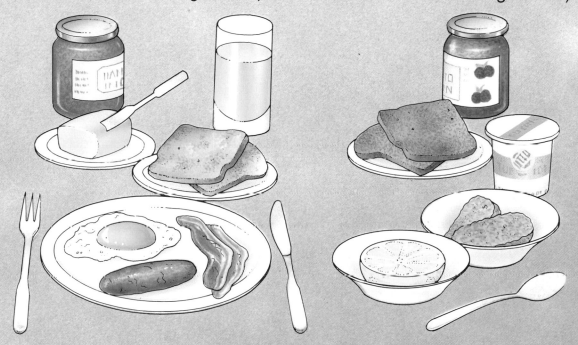

Most people eat around 20 g of fibre each day. **Experts** believe that people ought to increase the amount they eat to at least 30 g. Changing from a breakfast like the first, to one more like the second would be a good start.

If you want to find out how much fibre you ate for breakfast this morning, you will have to do some simple sums:

1. Find out how much fibre 100 g of each item you ate contains. Breakfast cereal packets make this quite easy. Look closely next time you are in a supermarket, and you will find that many labels tell you how much fibre (and other nutrients) are found in 100 g of the product. You can also use the list on page 26 to help you.

2. Weigh a normal helping of each item on some scales and note down the weight.

3. For each item, divide the weight of a normal helping into 100 g (this will tell you how many times smaller than 100 g your helping is).

4. Divide the weight of fibre contained in 100 g of the food by your last answer. This will tell you how much fibre a normal helping of the food contains.

For example:

A. 100 g of Weetabix contains 12 g of fibre
B. Normal helping of Weetabix = 50 g
C. 100 g ÷ 50 g = 2
D. 12 g ÷ 2 = 6 g of fibre in 50 g of Weetabix

To find out how much fibre the entire breakfast contained, add together the weight of fibre in each of the items.

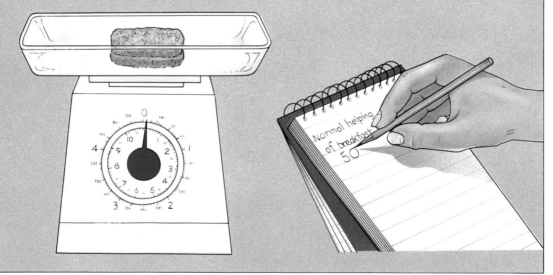

Bran contains more fibre than any other food on the list; fibre makes up nearly half of its weight. But bran is very light and 100 g is much more than most people would want to eat at once. To plan a high-fibre diet you have to think about how much fibre is contained in normal helpings of the foods you want to eat.

It is interesting to find out as much as you can about the food you eat. The more you know, the better you will become at choosing tasty, healthy food. Why not help to grow some of it if possible? Help to shop for it, asking lots of questions and looking at the labels. Help to prepare it and learn new recipes. But don't worry about your diet. If you make gradual changes towards the kind of food described in this book, there is no doubt you will be getting plenty of fibre, as well as all the other things you need to grow strong and healthy. Enjoy it!

BELOW Why not have a go at making your own personalized breakfast cereal, thinking carefully about how to make it healthy and tasty?

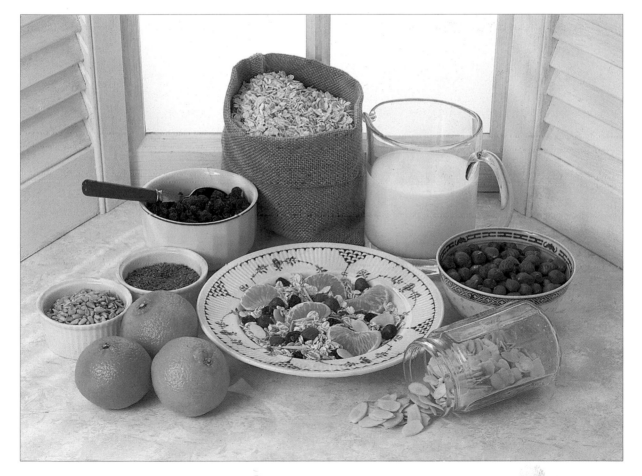

Glossary

Absorbed   To have taken something in.
Ancestors   People who lived long ago.
Bran   Part of the outside skin of cereals which contains a lot of fibre.
Cells   Tiny parts of living things, which we are unable to see with the naked eye.
Cereals   Edible grains, such as wheat and barley, and the foods made from them.
Constipated   Unable to go to the toilet.
Diet   All the food a person eats.
Digested   To have taken in what the body needs from the food eaten.
Digestive system   The parts of the body which are used to digest food.
Developed countries   Rich parts of the world, such as the USA or Europe.
Developing countries   Poorer countries of the world with little industry.
Experts   People who know a lot about a certain subject.
Extracted   Taken out.
Factory processes   A series of actions in a factory.
Industrial Revolution   A time of great change, when machines in factories took over from small scale work in homes and villages. It began in the early nineteenth century.
Knead   To pound and fold the bread dough.
Luxury   Something too expensive for everyday use.
Microscope   A special piece of equipment used to magnify tiny objects.
Nutrients   All the things in food that the body needs to remain healthy.
Organically grown   Grown using no poisonous sprays or artificial fertilizers.
Papyrus sieves   Sieves made out of a particular type of reed. They were used by the ancient Egyptians.
Poisons   Substances which can harm the body.
Texture   The feel of something, for example whether it is rough or smooth.
Yeast   Something used to make bread rise.

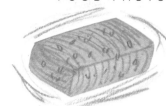

Books to Read

Food for Thought by Gill Standring (A & C Black, 1990)

Diet by Brian Ward (Franklin Watts, 1991)

Beans by Terry Jennings (A & C Black, 1990)

Fruit by Miriam Moss (A & C Black, 1991)

The Food Series (Wayland Publishers, 1989)

For Teachers

Bake your way to a better diet by Jane Inglis (Oakroyd Press, 1984)

Picture Acknowledgements

Aspect 9; Cash 11 (top), 22, 25; Cephas 20; Chapel Studio *Cover,* 5, 6, 8, 11 (bottom), 12, 15, 21; Bruce Coleman 7, 24; Jeff Greenberg 4; Tony Stone 19; Zefa 18, 29.

Index

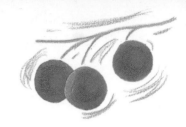